# Miracle of Acceptance

### Healing begins....

**Dr. S. Syed Jaffer**

**SSP Books and Digital Media**

Dedicated to my grandmother

Rabiya

# Table of the Content

# Preface

This book discusses the miracle of acceptance. How does it impact our life?

This book is the outcome of my spiritual journey from the age of 20. But I started my spiritual journey from childhood with my grandma. She planted the spiritual seed to my heart and her storytelling ability was mind blowing. She was blind from a young age. I learned lots of sufi and panchatantra stories from her. I am very grateful to my grandma. I dedicated this book to her wisdom. I never thought about this small book on spirituality.

In the first chapter, I discussed the belief system of our mind from a scientific perspective. Second chapter, how does thought form in the mind? The impact of thought in our daily life. Third chapter, you will see the image formation in the egoic mind and its consequences. Fourth chapter, you get the understanding of acceptance in life. Fifth chapter, you move more depth of acceptance from a sense perspective. Sixth chapter,  your immediate surroundings and their influence in your life. Parents, siblings, friends and relatives are your surroundings. How to accept them in your life?. Seventh chapter, your addiction and craving habits. How does it form in life? How to deal with them in real life?. Eighth chapter, your love for easily accessible things in life. Your mind always loves comfortable things. How to break a challenging dream into an easily achievable dream?. Ninth chapter, you go through the miracle of forgiveness. Then finally in the tenth chapter, you understand the true meaning of emptiness and its beauty.

I thanked my wife L.Saira Banu for her support and understanding. She helped in proofreading and valuable suggestions during the preparation of this book. I am grateful for her. I am thankful for my son's patience and understanding.

I enjoyed it a lot during the preparation of this book. Hope it will heal your life also. If you have any queries, feedback and suggestions about this book, then please write to us in **email: syedjaffer.s@outlook.com**.

This book comes through me, not from my efforts. Thank you very much.

Date: 03-11-2022                                        Dr. S. Syed Jaffer

Place: Coimbatore                                        (Author)

# About the Author

Dr. S. Syed Jaffer completed his PhD in chemical sciences from Indian Institute of Science and Education, Kolkata (IISER-Kol). He published good impact scientific papers in high rank international journals during his doctoral period. After that, he went to Seoul National University (SNU), South Korea for one year as a postdoctoral fellow in biophysical chemistry. When he returned to India, he joined as a senior scientist post in the industry for about six months. Currently he is working as an Assistant Professor in the department of chemistry, Coimbatore Institute of Technology(CIT), Coimbatore.

Recently, he invented a novel method to synthesize and process nanodiamonds and filed the same to an international patent agency ( WO2020115755A1, WO2020115754A1 ). Similarly, he invented novel amino acid based hydrogel from single molecular entities without any organic

solvent and polymers(WO2019021143A1, WO2019021144A1 ).

# 1. Introduction

We always live in two places in our entire life. You may wonder and be shocked about this statement. But this is our reality in this world. You may ask, "how is it possible?". First one is your physical reality, that is mainly the material world outside us. Second one is the nonphysical world, which is in our inside world. No one can see it! Hear it! Taste it! Smell it!. Even Though, it gets inputs from our physical senses. It is nothing but our own mind.

With the help of science and technology, we can control the outside world to a larger extent. Like, scientists made a very recent vaccine for the pandemic. It helped the countries to control and spread the virus. Today, with the help of artificial intelligence, corporate companies are running their marketing. In simple words, corporate companies know your likes and dislikes better than you. Last two centuries, we have achieved a lot in industries, science and technology in the outside world. Our achievements are only in the outside material world.

Yes, I agree, we are living in a beautiful, technologically advanced world as compared to a hundred years ago. We are enjoying the comfort of technology and science. Now the question is, "What is our achievement in the inside world?". Can you ask this question to yourself?. The answer for this question is " nothing". We achieved nothing in our inside world.

As mentioned, our inside world is our mind. Now the question is , "what is our own mind?". It is nothing but the collection of information and our own belief system. This information and belief system accumulated from our early childhoods. Teachers, parents, friends and siblings are the main feeder of these information and belief systems. Because you blindly trust them.

Are all human minds the same? Or is one person's mind different from another? The answer is yes. All human minds get thoughts in their brain.

The only difference between humans is the amount of thoughts. If the information is stored or recorded in your brain, then you will get a reflection of the information in your mind. These reflections of information are called thoughts. If these reflections of information move continuously in your mind as a chain, then it is called a thinking process. Here, this reflection of information operates in two ways. One reflection of information is superimposed with another reflection of information. That means, they are perfectly aligned with each other. Then you get blissing, joy, peace and happiness in your mind.

Next one is very complicated. It is called the enemy within you. Reflection of information is not superimposed with another reflection of information. They are not aligned with each other. This creates a continuous contradiction of thoughts. Then the person gets jealous, enmity, hate, negative emotions etc. These are the games of images. All these things are maya. It is the non true nature of our thoughts. That's it.

The same above said concept, we can discuss scientifically also. I tried to explain the concept of physics in layman terminology. This following upcoming explanation for non-science people. But, if you already know physics concepts also, then you will get a very new kind of insight in this subject. In physics, there are two types of branches. One branch deals with classical objects. Classical objects means big objects that you can see with your naked eyes. It is applied to big objects. The other name for classical physics is Newtanian physics. In this field, we have very well defined laws for nature.

Second branch is very busy with the objects that you can't see. Like , subatomic particles and photons go well with this branch. It is called quantum physics. It has gone well with Schrodinger equation, Heisenberg's uncertainty principle, and De Broglie's  duality theory for matter. Photon is another name for a light particle. You may ask, " Is it a light particle?". The answer is yes. According to classical physics, light is a wave in nature. But in quantum physics, sometimes light behaves like a wave and particle. It is the dual nature of small subatomic particles and light. Without light, seeing sense is not possible.

Light goes in all directions. There is no specific direction for light, except laser light. As mentioned earlier, light carries the information or message and it goes in all directions. How to make laser light? It is continuous excitation, emission, and reflection of light in between two mirrors. This process of operation gives unidirectional and single wavelength laser light (nearly). If you are in between the two mirrors, then you will get an infinite number of images of you due to an infinite number of reflections.

Thoughts in our mind also go into an infinite number of manifestations due to reflections and combinations. You can't control it normally. There are some yogic and kundalini techniques that you can stop thinking about. If you are in no thought by this root, then it will affect your normal life based on your previous karmas. It makes it difficult to do your daily activities. I, as an author of this book, not recommend and advocate for these techniques. That is not the scope of this book.

# 2. Thought comes in the mind

Another one more thought experimentation, If you place a single hole slit in front of light passage, then it makes no difference in light. But you do the same experiment with two hole slits instead of a single slit. It impacts a lot. What will happen now? We get diffraction fringes on the screen. It is bright with intense light and dark with no light. This is called diffraction fringes.

If light is perfectly superimposed with another light wave, then it gives a bright light spot. If light is imperfectly aligned with another light wave, then it gives a dark spot. It is called Young's double slit experiment. This operates very similarly like our thoughts.

Information and belief systems from our childhood are collected trash of our mind functioning. It is always a condition between our likes and dislikes and impacts us to see things as they are. You see the mind functioning of the child, which is totally different than well grown adults. Child brain has not grown fully yet. The information and the belief system of the child is limited. Child's brain neural network and neuroplasticity change very easily. They can adapt and accept new things or situations very easily.

But when you see a well grown and rigid brain of an adult, it won't accept any new things easily and not familiarize with new technological advancements. They are already so conditioned with their very strong false belief system. But unfortunately, everyone is  happy with these false belief systems. Now the question is ,"what is the belief system?" It is our near environment, the country we belong to, the religion we belong to, the basic food system we follow, and totally the cultural things we strongly believe in. In this, whatever we learned from the so-called educational system of school and college. Our parents, siblings, friends and teachers play a very important role in the belief system.

Now, we got the idea about the belief system. How does it develop and manifest in our life? It doesn't come overnight suddenly. It takes lots of days and years. These can be mainly categories as your likes and dislikes(hates). If you like ice cream, then you naturally love the conversation and information about the ice cream. Otherwise  you won't listen. Please note listening is one of the gifted sense among all senses that is given to humans.

If you see the beautiful scenery , then you lose yourself in that moment. Do you know the meaning of losing yourself? That is the beautiful moment in your life, you stayed without any thoughts. It is no thought state. This thoughtless state is nothing but gaps. Because you like good green scenery. Otherwise, you won't get a feeling of bliss at that moment. Seeing is another one of the gifted sense of nature.

Do you know the origin of these senses? There are five fundamental elements in nature. They are called sun, gas, space, earth and water. Without these elements, life is not possible on this earth. All living species have these elements in their life. They are not separated from each other. All of these elements are related to one another. But how? Prana is the vital force of life. We will discuss them later.

Do you know? Why do I put listening first and seeing sense second? There is a perfect reason for that. If you don't want to see anything, then you can close your eyes. That is a natural one. In this way, you can stop your seeing sense temporarily. But you can't stop your listening sense. Some of you may tell, by putting our finger in the ears. It is done by external influence. You can't stop listening naturally. Even it operates in your deep sleeping state, but you are not aware of that. There is no natural shutdown for listening. That is the reason I put it first.

These two are major senses for getting information in our daily life. But we have some more gifts like tasting, smelling, and touching senses. If something comes from outside and interacts, then these senses will activate and store the information in our brain. This information is stored inside our brain in the layer by layer and network link between the layers. Layer growth of the brain depends on the information received in daily life from parents, teachers, books we read, and people we interact with. The beauty of these layers, it's all connected with each other in an orderly manner.

If there is any mismatch or disorder in the network, then it causes stress or irritation in any situation. That leads to permanent or temporary confusion in their life. These networks do not work on a one to one basis. It works as one to many and many to one. For example, one good memory from any past experience is connected with your present memory or experience or information. All our likes or good memories are connected in one particular order. Similarly, all our dislikes or bad memories  are connected in another one particular order. We always expect good or likable memories from our life. It won't work like that. Life gives both good and bad memories. But how do you react to these memories or experiences? That decides your life destiny.

# 3. Egoic mind image formation

This order of likes and dislikes of our recorded memories or experiences gives birth to a new type of the entity. This new type of entity is your ego mind. 'I' word is another name for an egoic mind. We have so many layers of I's in our life. You are a son or daughter for your parents, this creates one type of 'I' layer in your mind with love and respect or hate and disrespect. That purely depends on your experiences or memories with your parents. You are a sister or brother for your siblings, this creates another type of 'I' layer in your mind as an image of good or bad. This 'I' depends on "how do they treat you in the course of life?". If your siblings give a lot of love and caring, then you give the same back. If you get any opposite from your siblings, then you also give back the same type of reactions to them.

Similarly, you make friends and colleagues in the outer layer of the family. You can choose your friends and teammates etc. But it is not possible in the family layer. If you like them or not, they are your parents and siblings. Whenever you make relation with the outer social layer of the world with someone, then what will happen?. Knowingly or unknowingly, you interact with their like and dislike layers. If you accept some of their likes or dislikes, then you make an outside network with people. We all are connected in this way, like your mobile or data networks. You can't see them physically. But they exist in your real life. These connections make a non-physical conscious world. That is the reason, if you meet some person in your life for the first time, then you get a good feeling about him or her. You make friends or good relations or choose a good partner for your life with the use of these non-physical connections.

This connection creates an image in your mind about that person or situation. If you encounter that person or situation in your life again, then you see them through this image only. You see him or her or any situation based on your past memories or experiences or images. It is easy for our brain. For the long run, this makes you dull as boring. You can't see any freshness in life. If you want freshness in your life, then you see things without past images. Is it possible in real life? Yes, that is what you will learn from this book.

You judge the person based on his past images or memories. If the image of the person or situation perfectly matches your belief system, then you like the person or situation. If the image of the person or situation does not match with your basic belief system, then you start to dislike or hate that person or situation without any reason. This process of building creates our collective ego mind. You believe this is your true state of the mind. It is our false ego created mind. If you trust your egoic mind, then it will take you down the wrong path.

But in our daily life, we need to trust and judge a person or situation. For example, we want to travel from one place to another place. First we need to plan our journey. In the process of planning, we should trust some of the things like the driving skill of the driver, people who work in the hotels or motels , and shopping places. Not judging means, accept the persons or situations without a single opinion about them or that in your mind.

Judgment is required for the outside world. But it is not required for the inner world of mind.

Take the example of bubbles in the sea shore,  you go to visit the sea shore. You can observe lots of  water bubbles there.  If you make a small little walk near them,then it hits on the feet and gives a chill feeling. After a short span of time, sea bubbles vanish without any effort from us. Then after some time a new tidal wave comes with similar bubbles. This will also vanish after some time. Nothing is permanent in this world. Change is the only unchangeable thing in this world. This is the rule of our physical world. But the problem is, one bubble strongly believes that it is bigger than other bubbles in the sea. But physically these bubbles are different in the size. But in reality, they all are bubbles. All of them vanish at the end.

 It is similar to comparing yourself with other people's skills. We all do not have the same strength physically. But we are human beings at the end of the day. Human being dies at the end without grabbing anything physically and even the knowledge accumulated through his or her entire life journey.

This is the truth and reality of life. You should accept it with a grateful heart.

With our own mind image of likes and dislikes, we always judge another person or situation. The word 'I' is nothing but our own likes and dislikes. If someone or situation aligns with our mind image of likes, then it is our good or feel better experience. If someone or situation aligns with our mind image of dislikes, then it is our bad or bitter experience in life.

# 4. What is acceptance?

Now, we are clear with our belief system. How is the belief system of the person related to acceptance? Let's put things in very simple terms. If someone or situation aligns perfectly with your mind image of likes, then you are in the state of acceptance. If someone or situation does not perfectly align with your mind image of dislikes, then you are in a state of nonacceptance.

State of acceptance of the mind is a good experience. Non acceptance state of mind is a bitter experience. Mind always loves to get good experiences in life. Mind expects to fill our life with good, loveable memories and experiences. This expectation creates lots of conflicts in your life. For example, you schedule your day with a short timetable. You expect to complete all the things 100% as you expected. Because of some other work, you are able to complete only 4o %. The remaining 6o% of work is still undone yet. In this your expectation is not fulfilled completely. Now I ask you one question, what will you do next? There are two options left for you. First one, you worry about not completing things at the time. Another one, you just accept it and move on to the next. The second one is the way of acceptance in life. You expect some good thing to happen in life. The output of any expectation is, it may happen or not. You should accept these two outputs in life. This is called acceptance.

Mind always fights with bad experiences in life. It tries to rebel or conflict with our thoughts. For Example, one person came and shouted very bitter words at you. Then you get angry and think about it day and night. Why did he shout at me without any reason? The outer bitterness comes after long storage of bad memories in life, you won't get an exact answer for these types of questions. You just accept the person and his bitter words and move on in your life.

Good and bad or likes and dislikes create images of our mind. The inner world, we fight between good and bad. Everyone wants only good in their life. No one wants bad in their life. But in nature, good and bad are the same. For example, top carnivores kill herbivores in the forest. According to you, top carnivores are bad. They are killing innocent herbivores. Top carnivores should kill herbivores for food and survival. It is the basic rule of nature and not bad. That we should accept.

Like floods, earthquakes, tsunamis, climate change, global warming and hurricanes are the product of nature. Nowadays we discuss these things in the media very frequently. They conduct hour long debates with some expert panel without any outcome. Yes, pollution and man made destruction are responsible for this. For survival, animals need only food and some place to rest. But humans need money for survival and to lead a comfortable life. Even top carnivores won't kill all the animals of the jungle. If they are hungry, then they go hunting. Otherwise, they just rest and play with others. Top Carnivores are very threatful animals in the forest ecosystem. But in real life, humans are more dangerous than them. We hunt every time. Even if it is not required also. Yes, we hunt for money. We should accept this.

Governments and big corporate organizations spend lots of money on infrastructure and business development projects. Today, business leaders decide on the government. That is the biggest disadvantage on democratic system. They destroy the forest and our beautiful ecosystem in the name of a developmental project. My intention is not putting anything against the developmental projects. We need all these things for sustainable development with the best ecosystem. For example, Japan created small forests in the city in the parking lane and high traffic areas. This removes most of the pollutants from the air. We need a good environment to live a good, healthy life. Bad environments and pollutants affect our senses and thoughts.

If you conflict and rebel with your own thoughts, then your conflicts magnify to a large extent. In simple terms, the acceptance diminishes the image formation of the mind. Non acceptance or conflicts magnifies  the image formation of the mind. Why does image formation in the mind affect our life? Once you form the image in your mind, then you start to see the person or situation through it. In this way of image formation of mind, we lose the freshness of life.  That is the reason, it is prohibited  in certain religions. In the Vedic tradition, it is called advaita.

Good and bad things will come to everyone's life. We can't stop it. We need to accept it. Acceptance is the solution for all problems. Like day and night, our mind runs from one extreme to another extreme. Please don't judge, day is good and night is bad. We are a living species. That is the reason, our mind moves. It shouldn't be in the static state. You can't stop your mind from moving. But there are some tantric, kundalini and breathing methods to control or stop mind movement. This is not the focus of this book. If you stop your mind movements, then you will be like a vegetable. In this case any one comes and uses you like a vegetable. Then you will not get any new ideas in life. Sometimes, it is difficult to do our daily activities. It is kind of dangerous for life. It is good for the people staying in the deep forest without any interaction with people.

But in real life, we need this beautiful working mind. It is for social interaction with people and to do our daily activities. In the next chapter, we are going to discuss acceptance in the sense level.

# 5. Acceptance from the senses

In the last chapter, we discussed the acceptance of the thoughts and belief systems. How thought forms its structure? Like computers, we feed information or command codes through the keyboard and by the internet. With these instructional codes, computers make some structural or functional outcome. Zero to one is very difficult in science and technological innovation. One to many is very easy. You will not get any permanent technology. Because everything is temporary in technology. It keeps addon.

Let's come to our question, thought is the beautiful thing. We can solve problems, construct bridges, houses, day to day activity etc by using our thoughts. What is the instruction code for our thoughts? Our senses are the instructional code for our thoughts. When the child sees something at first, he or she won't understand anything. Parents and teachers are the persons who feed the conditional instruction to the child. Some it gets from the outer social environment. Your thoughts depend on the environment and social-cultural background you belong to. Thought forms through seeing, listening, touching, smelling and tasting senses. According to vedic and yogic scriptures, if your senses are good and alive, then you will get a peaceful, happy, joyful and mindful life.

How is it possible? Some guru tells you to do yoga practice. Other gurus tell you to do intense meditation practice. Really you want all these things to get good senses. You do not need to do yoga and meditation practices. Like most people, they practice morning one hour and evening one hour for yoga and meditation. After that they go to work and do all the nonsense. In this way, is it possible to get good sense by doing all these practices? No, you will not get perfect sense from these methods. Because you will become more mechanical by the methods and practices. Mind always try to convert your practice or experience into mechanical or automatic mode. Then you see or observe or listen to things from your past memories. It is an easy and comfortable way for the mind.

Without all these practices, is it possible to see things freshly every moment? Yes, it is possible. As we discussed no use of any of these practices. If your life is a meditation, then you do not need separate meditation. Before proceeding further, you should know about concentration and attention. What is the difference between concentration and attention? Both are different from one another. Concentration is putting all your senses in the particular focus point. It is nothing but focusing your senses on a single point. This creates lots of stress on the person, who practices these concentration practices. Attention is totally or whole to observe something with your senses. It is just the opposite of your attention. In simple terms, concentration is the focus. Attention is defocus or non focus.

Among those two, which one belongs to meditation? Both are required, but one is essential. For example, if you work hard physically, then you can enjoy your rest time. You  go to the ground and play football for an hour. That time you should put full focus and concentration on the grounds. Then the game was over after an hour. This time you go to relax and defocus mode.  You feel happy even though you're tired. Focusing one thing for a long period of time, then you release your focus or defocus. This relaxes our body and mind, which gives you happiness. Concentration gives you stress. Releasing the concentration or defocus gives you happiness and joy. That means, attention is essential for meditation. Now the question is, "How to get attention without concentration?".

In your mind, you can sense one thing at one time. You can't sense seeing and listening at the same time. For example, you are looking outside in the rainy and lightning time. What will you see first? Sound or light. Light hits first and after some delay sound comes. We all are seeing by light. We all are listening by sound. Seeing comes first and then listening. According to neuroscientists, thought stays in the mind for about 15 seconds. Most of our thoughts are repetitive, it comes and goes. If we are able to increase the gap between the thoughts, then we can go to that source point of happiness and joy. You can increase the gap between the thoughts by staying with them. That staying with thought is called acceptance. If you fight or rebel with the thought, then it creates conflicts and more thoughts popup in the mind.

First we go to discuss seeing sense. If you are going to some crowded place, then you can see lots of people there. In that time, your mind is focused and seeing one particular person. That is called concentration or focus or separation of that person from the rest of the crowd. This way the mind manipulates our senses. Here, you are observing one person, not the entire crowd. You are not seeing the wholeness of the crowd. Is it possible to see the wholeness? Yes, it is possible for everyone. Observer is our recording mind, it wants to see the entire whole crowd. But your sense of seeing only recorded or observed one particular person, not the entire whole crowd. Here, observer is not equal to observed. That creates conflict between the observer(recording mind) and the observed(seeing sense). The recording mind collects and stores all the information about your entire life. Another name for this recording mind is your heart. This is not a physical heart. No need to confuse yourself, we will discuss in the upcoming chapter.

When we grow older, this conflict also grows with us. With the help of this particular function of the mind, we can study things, analyze, categories and classify. Our entire education system is focused on this basic fundamental concept. You need this mind function to study things. It is required for science and technology. It creates more disorder in our life. But you can't see or understand the beauty of the crowd by seeing one person.

If the observer is observed, then you will have perfect order and acceptance in the mind. You get this order in the night sleeping time. Sleep is the natural healer. Sometimes it is expressed as dreams. You can see some dreams in your mind during night time. The deepest layer of the dreams, you can't be aware. For example, in the physical world you desire any luxury car ride. It is difficult in the outside world. But it is possible in the dream. Now your desire is an observer and your dream is observed. Both are perfectly aligned. That is one of the reasons why dreams come to us.

In the state of "Observer is observed", that is the tiny moment you stayed in the presence moment. In this moment thoughts won't come into your mind. Your mind can't understand anything about this moment. It stays calm in that state. That you can name emptiness or gap. But it is a nameless state of mind. Their mind stops automatically without any effort. But it is a temporary one. You can enjoy these tiny presence moments of the mind

state.

# 6. Accept your parents, siblings, relatives and friends

We all come from our parents. Without them no one would exist here. I agree that some of you lived happily with your parents. Others passed through bad childhood experiences. If the parent treats you with lots of love and compassion, then you get a good experience in your life. It is quite obvious. Some of them abuse their child physically and psychologically. Why do parents abuse their childrens? They have lots of conflict and hate in their life. That they simply pass to their children.

If you are happy with your parents, then you accept them easily. Whenever you get their memories in life, then you feel happy and joyful. But that is not the case for everyone. For example, if any person's mother or father treated him very badly, then that person carries a very bad memory about them. Whenever he or she sees the photo or images of his or her parents in the outer world, he or she gets the thought image of them in their mind. If your experience with them is good, then it is a joyful one. If your experience with them is bad or abusive, then it makes you feel more hatred and suffering. Now the question is, "How to deal with this issue?". You ask yourself, "Who is asking to deal with this issue?. Your immediate answer is "I". That "I" is nothing but your egoic self of mind, that is nothing but your accumulated memories, knowledge, and experience from this life. With the egoic self of "I", you can't solve anything. This will increase your problems. That's it.

In the Holy Bible, they call Moses code. The statement is, "I am that I am". Similar statement in there in the ancient holy vedic scripture . The statement from the vedic text is, "Aham Brahmasmi". The approximate meaning of this beautiful vedic text is, "Creator resides in". In the Holy Quran, the same statement repeated as, "I am closer than your jugular vein". It is very close to us. But we lost in this world. How to find this? The first question is, "Can we live peacefully without this? No, you can't live without this peacefully in this world. If you name it, then you miss it. We came here in this world to just realize this and unite with the source. If you realize or unite with the source, then you succeed in this life. You do not need to go to the forest or any type of practice.

We all are already connected with this source. But you are unaware about that. If you are expecting something from the source, then you won't get anything from this. We get everything from this source only. "We won't get what we ask in the prayer. We get the things from what we are". You came from the source. Your parents also came from the same source. Everything in this world is connected to this source. If you are complaining or blaming your parents, then you are accusing the source for your life reality. In another way, if you accept your parents with fullness, then you are grateful for the source to this life. That simple act gives lots of peace, joy and happiness in your life.

You may ask the method for acceptance. I am repeating again, there are no methods or practices for this. For example, we try to run or escape from bad thoughts. We try to talk very much with other people, watch movies, waste time with unhealthy habits and do some intense workout. Some of us go into bad addictions.  Yes, you can escape from your thoughts by doing these. But it is not the permanent solution for the problem. If you keep quiet for sometime without doing anything, then the same bad thoughts will pop up in your mind.

You just stay with that thought and don't run or escape. You give your full attention for  that thought from all of your senses. Just wait without any expectation or outcome, you stay without judging, blaming and complaining. Any thought can't stay more than 15 seconds. When we convert thought into thinking, then it will stay longer. Now, the bad thoughts start to disappear slowly. Disappearance of the thought depends on the impact and depth of the thoughts. Some thoughts with the low impact disappear immediately. Some thoughts with medium impact disappear after days and months.  Some thoughts with deep impact disappear after years. The impact of thoughts depends on our attachment to the thoughts. If you are very much attached to your thoughts or things, then it creates a deep impact in our mind. If you have very shallow thoughts with almost nil attachment, then it creates a low impact in our mind. Healing takes time depending on the thought impact in the mind.

You can't choose your siblings. They are your siblings even if you like them or not. For example, we get natural light during the day from the sun. Here, the sun is the source of light. Light rays come from the sun. But light rays are not the sun. Each and every light rays are connected with the sun. Because they came from the same single source. Light rays carry the information about the sun. Each and every light rays are siblings. When it reaches earth, some light rays go and hit to give life to plants and some rays try to evaporate to form cloud cycles and  some rays just warm up our planet. In the same analogy, we all are connected with our source and carry the imprint of the source. You and your sibling do not carry the same amount of information and knowledge in this world.

This difference of opinion is required in the family. That you should accept completely without any hesitation. Then you can live peacefully with your siblings. Similarly, you can deal with your relatives. This is your family circle.

Now you can go to the outer circle of the work. Here, we make friends. It fully depends on our free will and choice. How do you make friends in life? If their mindset and believe system are aligned with yours, then you call them your friend. If it is not aligned, then you go just opposite. Choosing a partner also, we do in the same way. Your likes become their likes. Your dislikes become their dislikes. Two bodies physically with one thought. This is your false image. Same thought is not possible. If only one same thought is possible, then we get peace in every way of life. But the basic nature of the thought, it creates conflicts and differences of opinion. That is the reason, we are seeing so many breakups and divorces. Because they are not ready to accept reality, they love to live in a thought created imagination world. This imaginary world gives only suffering in life.

# 7. Accept your cravings and addictions

What is craving? Craving penetrates into our daily life from different sections and parts of the life. Now, we can see their influence in our life. Before, we go into detail discussion. We should know the basic mechanism of habit formation. Our good habits make our life well in all aspects  and our bad habits make life more destructive. Why do we need to separate habits as good and bad? Inner world of thoughts, we do not need to separate anything. We should accept everything in the inner world that gives us peace. But in the outer world, we need to deal with material things, work and relationships etc.

To deal with the outer world, we need separation. If the things or acts are harmful to you, then it is bad for us.  If the things or acts are good to you, then it is good for us. Habit formation is very essential for life. First you do a simple act. It creates memory in our brain cells and good feeling associated with it. Good emotion and feeling gives some neurochemicals. We have some neurochemicals with  good feelings and emotions.  That gives good memories in life. Whenever you get good memories, then your brain releases that neurochemicals. If you remember these memories, then you will get the same release of neurochemicals. It will trigger the same part of the brain.

Again and again, repeating the same acts or remembering that, it makes very strong memories in the brain. That forms a habit. If it becomes a habit, then you get these neurochemicals regularly. Because, your brain cells are like that.

We love to get only  good memories from life. But in reality, we get both bad and good memories. We all hate bad  memories and experiences in life. Why do the brain cells love good memories and experiences? It purely depends on our belief system. If your basic belief system loves good memories and experiences, then your brain cells like that. If your  basic belief system towards pain, sorrow, bad memories and experiences, then your brain cells like the same.

Animals eat food for hunger. It goes hunting to fulfill the hunger.
They have very little food choices. Their food varieties are also limited
in numbers. But you see, we have more varieties of food. We are
eating because we are not only hungry. We have so many food
varieties and their tastes are one of  the reasons for eating. As we
discussed earlier, these tastes of the food creates neurochemicals inside
our brain cells. Whenever you remember or see or feel that particular
food, then you will release the same neurochemical inside the brain.
That activates the particular region of the brain. It triggers craving in
the mind. How to deal with craving? We like to solve problems. You
can focus on the outer world to solve problems. You can't even solve
any single problem of the inner world. If you try to solve inner world
problems, then you will create more manifested problems in life.
Then, what to do now? Just keep quiet for some time. Everything
settles down as muddy water. For example, you take a packet of water.
Then you drop one small stone in that through the center. You can
see a lot of waves going from the center to the side and reflecting back

vice-versa. Now, you decide to stop these surface waves by putting your hand in it. As long as you try, you get more waves and disturbance in the surface water. But if you wait without doing anything for sometime, then these water surface waves stop naturally.

You no need to stop craving thought. If you try to stop craving thoughts, then you will get more craving thoughts in your mind. You just stay with your craving thoughts. It creates sensation in the body. No need to give your attention to the craving thoughts. You give your complete attention to the sensation in the body. You no need to translate or interpret or judge the sensation. Sometimes you get a strong sensation. Most of the time you have a very weak sensation. In some cases, you get an intense pain sensation in the body. Your job is just to stay with it without any judgment.

This craving goes off naturally, it takes time to heal. This is a natural process. If your body sensation is very intense, then it will take time to heal itself. You should accept your craving and wait to heal naturally.

If a person flows with craving, then that person will end up with addiction. For example, any person drinks a cup of coffee every morning. Because of some reason, you miss the morning coffee. If it does not affect your daily routine, then you are not addicted. If it does, then it is an addiction. You are not taking any coffee for the month. Then it is OK. You are not dependent on any substance. Most of the time, people fall back to addiction due to craving sensation in the body. You can replace the coffee with smoking cigarettes, alcohol, overeating, abusing any person etc.

Craving sensation of the body is responsible for addiction. The same craving sensation forms the habits in our daily life. It is linked with our belief system. For example, you love to read books daily. Those are good habits. But it depends on the type of the book you read. If you are not reading a book for some days, then you will not get any craving sensation in the body. That means, your mind is not urging you to read the book. You can stop it anytime and start anytime. That is a really good state of the mind. The opposite of this gives irritation and a craving feeling. This good habit is also an addiction. In this example, you can replace the reading book with other good habits such as walking, good diet, yoga, meditation, positive affirmation etc.

If you are missing these good habits rarely, then you should accept it with full of your attention. You don't need to be so rigid in your life. Let it go, that is the approach required for life.

# 8. Mind loves comfort zone

In physics, all particles travel from one place to another with the least path action. Earth rotating around the sun due to gravitational force. Earth takes the least path of action at that particular force. If you throw the ball, then it takes the least path of the action. This is the natural physical process. Similarly , our mind is like a comfort zone. What is a comfort zone? If someone asks you to go out and take a coffee, then it is an easy one for you. That is your comfort zone for coffee. But, if someone asks for a million dollars from you, then it is not easy. Now you are not comfortable with a million dollars. Your mind projected the image that coffee is easy and a million dollars is not easy.

It purely depends on your belief system with the things and situations. If you are a multi billionaire, then million dollars is very easy. That means, a billionaire is comfortable with a million dollars. In this way, we differentiate everything in our life. For example, water is a very essential substance for life on the earth. Without water,  it is very hard to live a life. It is available in abundance almost freely everywhere. But gold is not that essential thing for life. But we value gold rather than water. That is our reality. If anyone asks for a cup of water, then you will give it immediately. But, if someone asks for gold, then you run out. We all operate on our mind created images.

If you think the gold and million dollar is very difficult, then it moves away from your life as a distant thing or situation. "What you think that you become". You are nothing but your belief system. You can change your belief system with continuous affirmations. Things will manifest in your life, when that comes in your belief system.

Every one of us is moving in our own time-line. What is our life time-line? This present moment is your time-line. Most of us won't accept it. Because we stay with our past memories or events and are afraid or dream about the future. Your physical body is in the present moment. But our mind projected either the past and future. This is the common thing for everyone. The problem arises, if we stay more time in the past or future, then we get a stressful, problematic and suffering life. Author repeated the same statement again, "staying in the present moment is the only solution". Mind always tries to escape from the present moment. We should investigate first, "Why does the mind stay in the past or future moments?" Because it is comfortable in the past memories and future dreams.

Past memories tell stories in our mind. If the stories of past memories are nice to you, then you will enjoy it. That is your greedy state of mind. As mentioned, the mind tries to move to the extreme. After some time, If the stories of past memories are bad, then you will start to worry. That is your fear state of mind. Greed and fear are like a pedal in the mind on the present time-line. With help of past memories, we think about good moments of life that associate with greed and about sadful moments of life that associate with fear.

Similarly, our future dream is also telling stories in the present moment. Because you are motivated with a future dream. You dream about living in a beautiful nice villa,  going on vacation in the dream place, completing the dream project,  and writing a nice book. We have both online and offline motivators. These motivations from the motivators push you to do something in life. They indirectly preach to you, if you are not doing anything, then your life is useless. They always tell us, you try to get something out of this life. We all have only one life. That is now and here. You just try to live this life. We do not need to use this life. If you start living your life, then you start your life in the present time-line.

Achievements and dream fulfillment moments won't give you real happiness in life. Of course, it gives a comfortable life outside. But it causes more sorrow and suffering inside. I am not against any achievements and dreams, You can dream and achieve with the help of the present time-line. If you move away from  the present time-line, then you get all stressful things in life even if you achieved your dreams.

As I discussed earlier, the mind tries to move out from the present time-line. For example,  you want the new beautiful dream house for you and your family. This is your long dream. Now , you are living in a small, narrow, bad piping and old dirty color wall house. You hate your current house and at the same time, you dream for your new beautiful house. You are staying in two extremes. On one side, you are expecting a new beautiful house and on the other side you are blaming and complaining about your current house. House is the common thing. One type of house you love and another type of house you hate. "Love and hate can't travel in the same boat". If you are in this state, then your dream will not come true in this lifetime. What next?

If you want your dream beautiful house, then you should be grateful for your current house. That means, you are accepting your current house. You are thankful for this current from the core of your heart. In this moment of gratitude to your current life situation, you come automatically into your present time-line without effect. At that time of gratitude, you dream of a beautiful house with a swimming pool etc. You try to visualize your dream like that you already had everything in your life. Like, you are walking through the green garden and touching the leaves. You enter the hall and switch on the smart TV and watch movies online with comfort sitting. First and foremost thing is, you should be comfortable with your visualization. Your mind feels comfortable with this visualization. If your mind is not comfortable with the visualization, then it throws away that from your life. Whatever you are wishing, expecting and praying in life, that is not important. If your mind is comfortable with it in the present time-line of gratitude, then your wish will be fulfilled naturally without any effort.

There is only one simple way, you can make anything comfortable. You should be thankful to everything that you have in this life. You should be grateful for your health, wealth, knowledge and the people around you. You think and visualize your dream daily at least 10 times. You believe from the heart, "that is easy". Because the mind loves easy things in life. If your mind tells you that it is hard, then you break your hard dream into small believable dreams.

Your target dream is a beautiful house at the cost of 0.5 million dollars. Now you are earning $50K per annum. You're saving around 30% of the salary. At the end of each year, you get around $15K in the bank. Then you invest your savings in best government bonds, IRS, mutual funds, ETFs and high dividend growth shares. If your investment grows by 8 to 15 % every year with compounding, then you will have around 0.2 million dollars in the bank account. Then you can easily get a bank mortgage to buy a nice house. In this calculation, your salary increment for every year is not calculated. Sometimes, job shifts also give 35 to 60 % hike in the annual income. This logical story for your dream house, you should try to convince your mind. If the mind starts to believe these stories without any single doubts, then you will get miracles in your life. You may ask, "What to do if doubt arises? As I discussed earlier, the mind tries to move in two extremes. Sometimes the mind believes in your story, after sometime it pops up some doubts on the same story. Gratitude is a basic thing, which naturally takes off the doubts from your mind. First type of gratitude is things you possess in life . Second type of gratitude is that other people pay you. One is giving gratitude and another one is receiving gratitude. This makes your life meaningful. Giving gratitude is a very normal one. But receiving gratitude makes your life meaningful. If more people become grateful to you, then you are a very famous person or celebrity. How many people's lives are you going to touch in a good way? That makes you.

For  example, you want a good management degree from a very famous institution in the US. If you dream day and night in your entire life, then you won't get anything. You need an action plan. First thing, you should go to a good school and get a better grade. Follow the best method for cracking the entrance test. If you have one year for the preparation, then you break the preparation plan into small daily and easy weekly schedules. You cross check daily your activity. Because your mind is comfortable with easy and small things.

Don't give that much importance to your dream and things. At the same time, you convince your mind that it is very easy. Then you will get them in life. You don't expect anything. Because, your expectation creates the importance of that thing or dream in your mind. Then the dream or things moves away from the present time-line due to the extra importance. How do you achieve anything without giving importance?

If you are dreaming of going to the star hotel for dinner everyday, then you will be normal and comfortable after sometime. Immediately, you get thought about money. If you have enough money, then it is normal and comfortable for you. In reality, you have little amount in the bank for survival for the next few months. Then it creates a strong doubt in your mind about money. You can't fake your mind and senses. But we all have gifted things in our life. That is our imagination. If you imagine now about your choice of tasty food, then you observe more saliva in the mouth. Just visualizing something won't give anything. It is similar to watching movies the whole day in your mind.

If you visualize with the senses and comfortable present time-line, then the miracle of acceptance flows in your life.

# 9. Miracle of forgiveness

Life doesn't give comfort, health, knowledge and wealth for everyone. Everyone's life is unique and different. Their core dreams and life desires also vary depending on the environment and surroundings. Most of the time, we try to compare ourselves with other people like he got a very nice house and had a good career. But you are not having your own house and permanent job etc. These types of comparison thoughts give jealousy in life. Whom do you compare? We compare ourselves with our loved ones and enemies. If your father or mother is a multi-millionaire, then society expects the same from you. Because society believes, you try to follow in his or her footsteps. That means, you are moving away from your present time-line. This act of following someone creates more stress and sorrow in life. Who is responsible for this suffering and sorrow? Of course, your parents are not responsible for that.

That is your own belief and your agreement with the society's belief system. Society is nothing but people. The people who are achievers in society, very few. You can take a list of people who are famous for their work in any field of life. Other people just do the facilitators job. They work for the government, teachers, corporations and big industries.  Generally, you get more openings in facilitators jobs. It is quite easy compared to building your own empire. That's how society preaches you everytime. Making from zero to one is very difficult. But you can create one to many very easily. From the above statement, if your belief system aligns with "making from zero to one", then you are an innovator or person for a new startup or creator in any field.

If your current belief system aligns with "making from one to many", then you are the best manager or facilitator or administrator. What is your belief system? Your belief system aligned well with administration. But you want to become an innovator. Then finally, you get only failure. That is the truth. "Nature won't give what you wish, it gives what you are". First you should forgive the people, whoever is expecting something from you. Why? For example, your parents expect you to become a football player. They put you in intense football coaching from childhood. But, if you have no passion for playing and like only watching, then that is not your belief system. But your parent tortured you to fulfill their dream. You do not need to fulfill their dream. Just accept that they tortured you. In this way you can forgive your parents.

The friend and society are expecting from you. For example, your friend is calling you to go out. But you are very tired and your mind is telling you to take rest. You like your friend and don't want to break the bond. He enjoys visiting places. But you don't. These type adjustments to the relationships, making you more away from the present time-line. That means, this so-called friend causes more suffering in your life. You should accept this fact. If you want to live peacefully, then you should forgive him or her. How to forgive anyone?

We remember everything in our mind, whenever you are remembering any life event. For example, you are watching football on the TV. Sometimes your childhood memories pop up. You get the painful and torturing image of your parents. They tortured you to go for the football coaching. You stay with the mind image of your parents with full attention. If you stay with the painful mind image, then you start to forgive your parents. Healing takes its own time depending on the impact of suffering. After some time, you start to accept your parents. This acceptance is the miracle of forgiveness.

You don't run from the painful memories, you just stay with it. You need to give your complete attention with full sense perception. Sometimes these painful memories give intense pain in some parts of the body. It varies from person to person, some cases get a fast heartbeat and breathing difficulty. You get these types of pain and abnormalities. That time, it is better to go to the psychologist or any therapist.

If you are not forgiving the people who cheated you, then you will be stuck in that moment. Forgiveness releases you from that moment. For example, your best friend cheated you for money or promotion. Then you get a painful memory about him/her. Why did he/she cheat me? This sequence repeats again and again in the mind. It gives more worry and sorrow in life. You do not need to investigate the reason for the cheating. You accept fully that he/she cheated me and stay with your complete attention. This miracle of acceptance gives healing from the pain and sorrow.

Now, we come to your enemies. Why do we have enemies? Because our mindset is not the same. Here, our focus is not the formation of enmity. We focus more on forgiving your enemy. If you do not forgive your enemy, then they occupy your mind space most of the time. That wastes your good time. They push you in your life. For example, you got a degree from a reputable institution. Now, you are going for a job as a fresher. If you are more intelligent than your peers, then most of the people from that team become your enemy. It comes from an evil jealous quality. They always wait for the chance to attack you. They gossip about you and try to create a bad name in the organization. Finally, you are fed up with them and quitting the job. This makes some changes in your life. It takes you to a good job or starting your own business. Now you see, enemies are required for growth. Pharaoh was required for Moses. Ravan was required for Rama. Kavravas were required for Pandavas.

Your enemies give negative energy to you. It is your job to convert their negative energy into positive. Here, positive affirmation gives more energy in our day today life. In this space, we all connected in a conscious way. Your consciousness is not different from the consciousness of the universe. These all are connected as one. It's another name is observer. In the real physical world, we have observers and observed. These two give us experiences and sensation in life. Our mind is observed. Because the mind consumes everything from the senses and translates. But our observer is very silent and doesn't do anything. It is just silent and sits there always. Even it won't interfere. Every day our mind dances different plays on it. But it keeps silent. The observer is called a heart. This is not a physical heart.

In the bible, "When your mind and heart is one. If you tell the mountain to move, then it moves apart". In vedic scripture, " Sat Cit ananda". The meaning is, "Sat" is the mind interpreted truth, "Cit" is the silent plain background of the mind and "ananda" is happiness, a product of perfect combination of Sat and Cit . Sufi mystical path of Islam, " Purify your heart is very essential to be near your creator".

# 10.  Miracle of emptiness

This is our final chapter of the book. We discussed a lot of things together in this book. Emptiness is the real goal of anybody's life. It is with us every time. But we are so busy in our mind activities. Why do minds occupy us? Because it masks the present time-line. From wake up to sleep, our mind makes us busy with a sequence of thought or overthinking. Your thoughts can't be an observer. Thought takes the form of an observer. Real observer that is inside of you won't say anything in life. It won't guess or judge anything. It stays with you in your good times as well as bad times. Then the mind asks immediately, What is the use of his observer? Without any expectation or use, Why do you stay with that heart?

Your mind takes you in the wrong directions. But if your mind is perfectly aligned with your heart, then the truth is revealed to you. Mind is full of knowledge and the heart is full of compassionate wisdom of love. How do they mix or combine? That is nothing but, "observer is observed". You and everyone is a formless consciousness being. Thoughts take the forms in the background of consciousness. If the thought vanishes in the background of consciousness, then you get emptiness. It is not loneliness. Emptiness is the perfect state of our conscious being. In this state, you will be connected or united with everything. How to get this perfect state of being? Almost all religious and spiritual teachers pointed out this.

We want this permanently. It is not a material thing. You can't hold it for the entire time. If you chase it, then it goes away from your life. If you keep quiet for sometime without any expectation, then it encapsulates your life with its wings. How to stay without any expectation in life? We always desire and expect something in this life. That is the basic nature of mind.

This is only possible with meditation. Generally, people do meditation in the morning and evening for half an hour. Then the rest of the day, they will do all the stressful activity without mindfulness. Meditation is not practice. It is the way of life. This gives awareness about you and your surroundings. For example, if you are going from one place to another place by walking, then you walk slowly and mindfully. Meditation is nothing but bringing attention in daily activities. Your feet touch on the ground, you just watch the sensation in the feet with full attention. Then you go for the next step. During this entire time, don't be in a hurry. You do it fully with complete attention. This is called walking meditation.

While doing work or job, you try to bring complete attention to the job or work. We already discussed that attention is different from focus. That means, you are doing your work or job outside. At the same time, your attention is on the senses of the body.  Because you get information about the outside through senses of the body. These observations create sensation in the body. Some of them, you can sense it due to intense. Other, you can't sense it due to its subtle effect. This sensation of the body is your observer or heart. This is responsible for your feelings and emotions. Like your mind grows when you age with information and knowledge. The same way, your heart grows with your bodily sensation.  When you are a kid, certain hormones are not there in the body. That time, if any beautiful girl or smart boy crosses to you, then you won't get any sensation. Because, your body is not ready for that type of sensation. Now, you enter your hot teenage days. You behave in a totally different manner for the above situation. Your body sensation goes up with increased heart beat and fast breathing. This is a very normal thing.

If you go to any Buddhist meditation center, then they ask you first to sit without doing anything. It goes for long hours. You mind chatting with lots of stories to move out. If you listen to it chatting without reaction, then it vanishes. After some time, the mind disturbance comes to an end. A Buddhist monk or master won't talk or explain too much like our university teachers. They simply watch you very closely. Your mind calms down. Then your sitting will be beautiful. You sit for long hours without any moment of the body. That is the first step, your mind accepts your sitting method. We all exchange our breath with our environment knowingly or unknowingly. We breathe. That is essential for life. You are not making any effort to breathe. It is happening very naturally. You know, we have two things in our breathing. We breathe in to take oxygen and breathe out to remove carbon dioxide. These things, everyone knows. There is a mystical thing in this process. During the inhalation, air goes through your nose and fills your lungs and stays there. After some time, it will come back as an exhalation to remove carbon dioxide from your lungs. This retention time between breathing in and out is called gap. If you have more gaps in the breathing process, then you are in a state of emptiness or happiness. This should happen naturally. This is called breathing meditation or Anapanasati. There are some techniques, you can do it with more practice. That technique is called Pranayama. Here, the person should control the breathing process.

One more addon is here. You can't watch your breath. Because breathing is formless. Your senses can't perceive any formless things. You're observing or watching the sensation in the nose when air touches it. When you breathe in, you get one type of sensation in the nose tip. When you breathe out, you get another type of sensation in the nose tip. During the breathless state, you have no sensation in the body. You can increase retention time naturally. But you can't make it permanently.

After the breathing sensation, you will go to see the body sensation. If you compare your body sensation with breath, then breathing is very normal. Because body sensation is your heart and observer too. It is an accumulated sensation of the body from your childhood. Sensation of the body is nothing but vibrations. Our physical heart beat is also vibration. Different emotions and feelings, your vibration of the sensation of the body varies. For example, if you are in the intense emotion of anger, then your body starts to vibrate. The words come from the mouth wimbles. The atoms and molecules vibrate, making them different from one another. Each atom vibrates at a different electronic energy level. Similarly, molecules are formed due to the bond between the atoms. These bonds also vibrate. Each molecule shows unique vibrations. We are all made by molecules physically. You can't translate the sensation to the normal worldly languages.

Each word of the language creates the image in the mind. We are the only living species that speak language. That language allows us to communicate with each other. But the same language creates confusion and conflicts. For example, you don't know chinese. If someone shouts at you in Chinese, then you won't get angry. Because you don't understand that language. But, you get some from their emotions and feelings. These emotions and feelings are  the universal language.

Now come back to the Buddhist meditation center, they ask you to watch the body. You try to observe the body sensation. If the sensation is there, then you just accept and acknowledge it.  Sometimes it won't show any sensation. That is perfectly OK. You just accept, it is not there. Then move on to other parts of the body. No need to analyze your body sensations and emotions. You just stay with it and accept it. After some time, you get no sensation. This sensationless state is called emptiness. Because we need thought to observe the body sensation. Without feeling and emotions, your heart becomes full of consciousness. Another name for this emptiness is total consciousness. Your consciousness is similar to the consciousness of another human. Not only that, your consciousness is connected with universal consciousness. The miracle of emptiness comes in your life without effort.